T0103514

HANDBOOK OF INTERVENTIONAL CARDIAC PROCEDURES FOR JUNIOR CARDIOLOGISTS

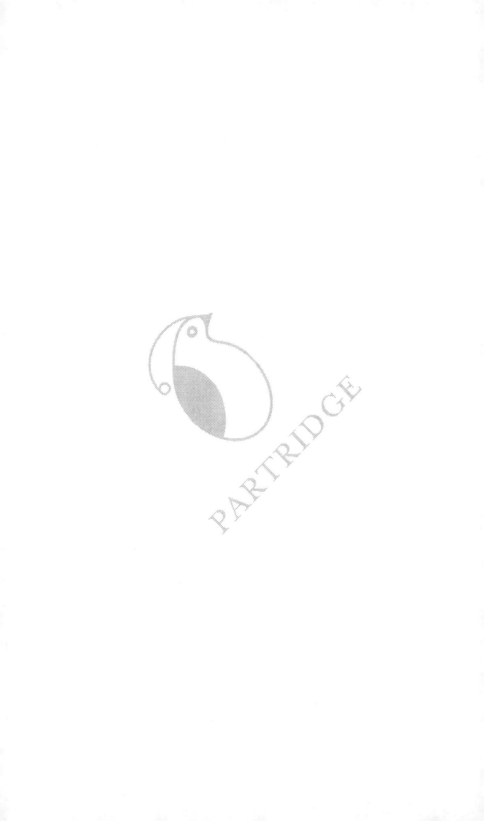

HANDBOOK OF INTERVENTIONAL CARDIAC PROCEDURES FOR JUNIOR CARDIOLOGISTS

(a summary of current cardiology literature)

Dr. Yahya Kiwan

Consultant Interventional Cardiologist
MRCP, FRCP, FRACP, FACC, FSCAI

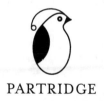

PARTRIDGE

To order additional copies of this book, contact
Toll Free 800 101 2657 (Singapore)
Toll Free 1 800 81 7340 (Malaysia)
orders.singapore@partridgepublishing.com

www.partridgepublishing.com/singapore

Table of Contents

1. Diagnostic Coronary Angiogram (CAG) 1

2. Transseptal Left Heart Catheterisation (TLHC) 5

3. Endomyocardial Biopsy (EMB) 8

4. Pericardial Intervention (PI) 11

5. Percutaneous Alcohol Septal Ablation (ASA) in Hypertrophic Obstructive Cardiomyopathy... 15

6. Percutaneous Transluminal Coronary Angioplasty (PTCA) 22

7. Mitral Balloon Valvuloplasty (MBV)..30

8. Pulmonary Balloon Valvuloplasty (PBV) 35

9. Aortic Balloon Valvuloplasty (ABV) 37

10. Transcatheter Aortic Valve Implantation (TAVI) 39

11. Transcatheter Mitral Valve Interventions 45

12. Percutaneous Closure of Paravalvular Leaks (PCPVL)..................49

13. Percutaneous Closure of Atrial Septal Defect.............................53

14. Percutaneous Closure of Patent Foramen Ovale (PFO).................56

15. Percutaneous Closure of Ventricular Septal Defect (VSD)............59

16. Left Atrial Appendage Occlusion (LAAO) 62

17. Coarctation of Aorta (CoA) 65

18. Carotid Artery Stenting (CAS)...69

19. Renal Artery Stenting (RAS) 75

20. Renal Artery Sympathetic Denervation (RSD)..............................80

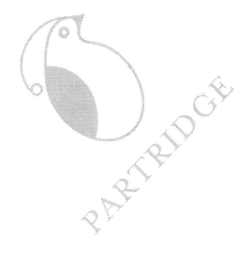

Author's Biography

- ## Qualifications:

MBChB	Iraq, 1977
MRCP	London, 1985
FRCP	Glasgow, 1997
FRACP	Australia, 1999
FRCP	UK, 2001
FSCAI	USA, 2002
FACC	USA, 2006

Experience:

1. One of the pioneers in the field of interventional cardiac procedures, Chest Hospital, Kuwait, 1985-1990.
2. A pioneer in interventional cardiac procedures at Charles Nicolle Hospital, Tunis, Tunisia, 1991-1995.
3. One of the pioneers in interventional cardiac procedures, Dubai Hospital, Dubai, UAE, 1995-1997.
4. Senior consultant interventional cardiologist in New Zealand and Australia, 1997-2006.
5. One of the pioneers in interventional cardiac procedures, Gold Coast Hospital, Gold Coast, Queensland, Australia, 2005.
6. Senior consultant interventional cardiologist, and in charge of the non-invasive cardiac laboratory at Dubai Hospital, from 2006-2011. Also senior lecturer at Dubai Medical College for Girls.
7. One of the founders of UAE intervention working group in 2010.

8. Currently senior consultant and head of department of cardiology, Canadian Specialist Hospital, Dubai, UAE.

9. Proactively involved in teaching and lecturing, as well as chairing a number of cardiac conferences at both the national and international levels.

10. As a recognised authority in cardiology, Dr. Kiwan has served as a subject matter expert for various publications and journals.

11. Currently serving as a subject matter expert for various cardiology publications and preparing his second book on cardiac interventional and surgical procedures.

ykiwan@yahoo.com
www.yahyakiwan.com

Reviewers

1. Professor Horst Sievert
Director of the Frankfurt Cardiovascular Centre, Frankfurt, Germany

"This book summarises, in a very clear format, all the basic information fellows and junior cardiologists need to know about cardiovascular interventions.

It reflects the tremendous experience of the author, Dr. Yahya Kiwan, whom I have known for more than 25 years.

For each procedure, the purpose, the indications and the contraindications, as well as the potential complications, are listed.

References are given for those who want to know more."

2. Professor JM Muscat–Baron,
Clinical Dean, Dubai Medical College For Girls, Dubai, UAE

"This is an excellent little book on the various diagnostic and therapeutic maneuvers that are available for interventional cardiologists.

It lists all the available procedures, the occasions when they are indicated, the hazards that may be encountered and provides a means to assess the results.

It forms an excellent introduction to the ever-expanding area of cardiology for junior staff interested in specialising in this field of cardiology.

Dr. Yahya Kiwan

3. Dr. Obaid AlJassim, MD, PhD

Cardiothoracic surgeon, Consultant and Head of Department of Cardiac Surgery, Dubai Hospital, Dubai, UAE

This is an excellent handbook on cardiac interventions, which I read with pleasure.

I found it extremely helpful, with practical ideas in intervention cardiology specifically written for junior fellows, although more senior ones would also find it useful.

Clinical chapters are very well organised and thoroughly address practical dilemmas, some of which are not well addressed, even in major textbooks! The readers get clear and direct tips on practical points to remember, learning indications, contraindications and possible complications for each procedure easily.

The information in this book is clear, outlined and well referenced. The chapters on transseptal left heart catheterisation, percutaneous transluminal coronary angioplasty, mitral balloon valvuloplasty, aortic balloon valvuloplasty, transcatheter aortic valve implantation, transcutaneous mitral valve repair, coarctation of aorta, renal artery sympathetic denervation and many other chapters are simply outstanding. The author seems to have a thorough grasp of the subjects and is well-versed in the latest trials in the field of cardiac intervention.

I have no hesitation in recommending this book to all junior cardiology fellows, and also the more senior fellows, residents and even general practitioners.

X

4. Dr. Abdulla Shehab,

Associate Professor and Consultant Cardiologist, UAE University, Al Ain, UAE

"The book style is concise and to the point, with a successive, logical flow of information.

I have enjoyed reading the book, and I would recommend it for junior cardiologists as a useful reference."

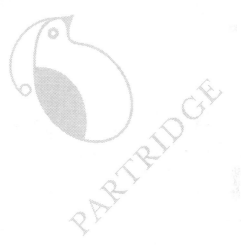

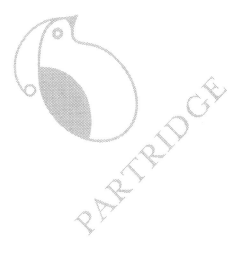

Very special gratitude to my mentors

1. Professor Giri Endrys
2. Proessor Abdulmohsin Al-Abdulrazzak
3. Professor Horst Sievert
4. Professor Naser Hayat

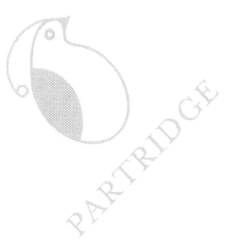

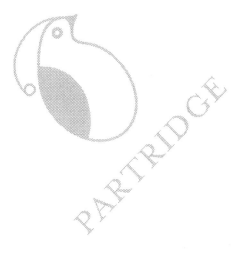

Acknowledgements

I am very thankful to my wife Ikram for her time and patience during my continued involvement in writing this book.

I am also appreciative of the work done by Dr. Nazish Ijaz for her active role in the preparation of the manuscript.

I would like to extend my thanks to my colleagues, mentioned by name in the list of reviewers on the previous page, for their valuable comments and input.

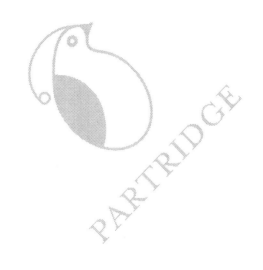

Preface

This book is published for doctors, especially juniors, working in all specialties of cardiology (clinical, non-invasive and invasive).

It is an up-to-date, practical, and user-friendly book that contains almost all the information needed by cardiologists in their day- to-day clinical work.

It derives its contents from the latest international cardiology guidelines and practices, and the most recent literature in the specialisation.

I am sure cardiologists of all different experience levels will find it useful.

I welcome your comments and feedback.

Dr. Yahya Kiwan
Dubai,
October 2015.

ykiwan@yahoo.com www.yahyakiwan.com

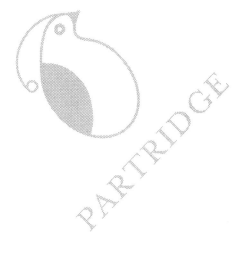

Abbreviations

	A
ASD	Atrial septal defect
AVR	Aortic valve replacement
AF	Atrial fibrillation
ASA	Alcohol septal ablation
ABV	Aortic balloon valvuloplasty
AV fistula	Arteriovenous fistula
AV	Atrioventricular
	C
CT	Computed tomography
CABG	Coronary artery bypass graft
CoA	Coarctation of aorta
CAS	Carotid artery stenting
CEA	Carotid endarterectomy
CCA	Common carotid artery
CAD	Coronary artery disease
	D
DVT	Deep vein thrombosis
	E
EMB	Endomyocardial biopsy
	F
FFR	Fractional flow reserve
	H
HOCM	Hypertrophic obstructive cardiomyopathy
	I
IVUS	Intravascular ultrasound
ICA	Internal carotid artery

	L
LVOT	Left ventricle outflow tract
LAA	Left atrial appendage
LV	Left ventricle
LAD	Left anterior descending
LBBB	Left bundle branch block
	M
MR	Mitral regurgitation
MVR	Mitral valve replacement
MBV	Mitral balloon valvuloplasty
MS	Mitral stenosis
MVA	Mitral valve area
	N
NOAC	New oral anticoagulant
NSTEMI	Non-ST elevation myocardial infarction
	O
OCT	Ocular coherence tomography
	P
PCI	Percutaneous coronary intervention
PFO	Patent foramen ovale
PCPVL	Percutaneous closure of paravalvular leak
PVL	Paravalvular leak
PPC	Percutaneous pericardiocentesis
PTCA	Percutaneous transluminal coronary angiography
PBV	Pulmonary balloon valvuloplasty
	R
RV	Right ventricle
RAS	Renal artery stenosis
RSD	Renal sympathetic denervation

	S
STEMI	ST elevation myocardial infarction
STS	The Society of Thoracic Surgeons
SAM	Systolic anterior movement
	T
TAVI	Transcatheter aortic valve implantation
TMVR	Transcutaneous mitral valve repair
TOE	Transoesophageal echocardiogram
	V
VT	Ventricular tachycardia
VSD	Ventricle septal defect

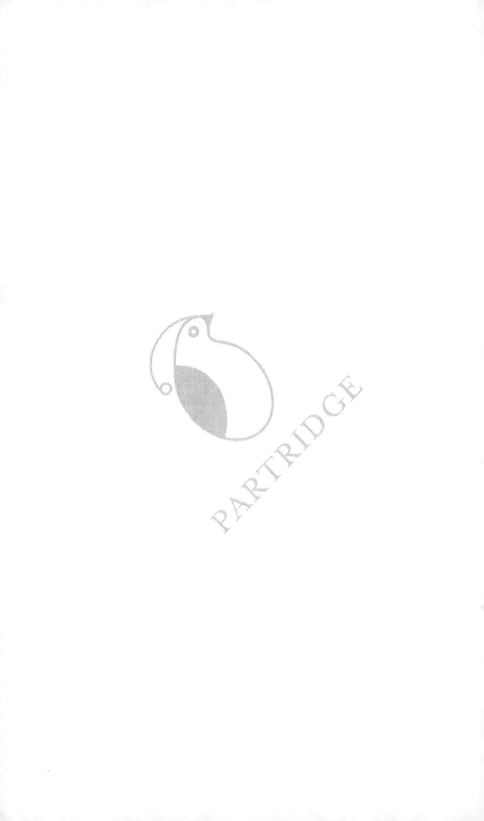

Classification of Recommendations and Levels of Evidence

Class of Recommendation	Levels of Evidence
Class I (strong)	Benefit >>> Risk The procedure or treatment (is recommended, indicated, useful, effective, beneficial) and should be performed or administered
Class II a (moderate)	Benefit >> Risk IT IS reasonable (can be effective, useful, beneficial) to perform the procedure or to administer the treatment
Class II b (week)	Benefit > Risk The procedure or treatment may be considered, might be reasonable, usefulness is uncertain
Class III: No Benefit (moderate)	No Benefit The procedure or treatment is not recommended, not useful not effective, not indicated and should not be performed
Class III: Harm (strong)	Risk > Benefit harmful and should not be performed

Levels of Evidence	
Level A	Data derived from multiple randomised clinical trials or meta-analyses of RCT
Level B	Data derived from a single randomised trial or non-randomised studies
Level C	Only consensus opinion of experts, case studies, or standards of care

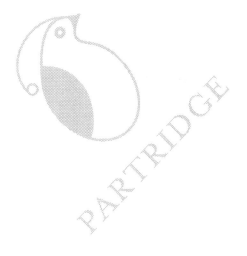

Diagnostic Coronary Angiogram (CAG)

Indications:

1. Patients with severe exertional angina.
2. Patients with positive non-invasive stress test.
3. Patients with suspected coronary artery disease, with inconclusive tests including **CT** coronary angiogram (as a diagnostic test).
4. May be considered as a preoperative preparation for major non-cardiac surgery in patients with known coronary artery disease.
5. As a semi-urgent procedure in patients with unstable angina or **N-STEMI**.
6. As an urgent procedure in patients with **STEMI** for a primary **PCI** or rescue **PCI**.

Contraindications:

- No absolute contraindications.

Relative contraindications:

1. Ongoing infections.
2. Severe anaemia.
3. Active bleeding.
4. Severe electrolyte imbalance.
5. Severe comorbidities.
6. Advanced age.

Aims (advantages) of coronary angiogram:

1. To determine the coronary anatomy, and any coronary anomalies.
2. To determine the location and severity of the coronary artery stenosis.
3. To determine the complexity of the stenosis (length, eccentricity, bifurcation, presence of calcification, thrombus or dissection).
4. To determine the physiological significance of the coronary stenosis (by using FFR, IVUS or OCT).

Complications:

While very rare, complications can take the following forms:

1. Access site complications:
    # Femoral approach: (2-5%)
      These include:
      1. Haematoma.
      2. Pseudoaneurysm.
      3. Arteriovenous fistula.
      4. Arterial thrombosis and distal embolisation.
      5. Retroperitoneal haematoma.
      6. Arterial dissection.
    # Radial approach:
      1. Total radial occlusion. (1-4%)
      2. Large haematoma.

2. Allergic reaction to contrast agent and potentially anaphylactic shock.

3. Hypotension: vasovagal or drug-induced.

4. Cardiac arrhythmias.

5. Pulmonary edema.

6. Myocardial ischemia and infarction due to:
   1. Contrast injection.
   2. Coronary thrombus dislodgement.
   3. Air embolism.
   4. Coronary dissection.

7. Stroke (0.1%-0.2%) due to thromboembolic events from:
   a) Access site sheath.
   a) Guide wire.
   b) Catheter.
   c) Plaque from the aorta.
   d) Thrombi from left ventricle.

8. Death: (0.1%)

Limitations of coronary angiogram:

1. Lack of adequate information on the correct type of revascularisation strategy. (**PCI** or **CABG**).
2. Limited data on plaque composition. (Requires invasive direct coronary imaging).
3. Cannot provide enough information on the physiological severity of the lesion (Requires the use of FFR).

References:

1. Judkins MP et al. Prevention of Complications of Coronary Arteriography. Circulation, 1974; 49:599
2. Baim DS. Grossman's Cardiac Catheterisation. Philadelphia: Lippincott Williams and Wilkins, 2006.
3. Percutaneous Interventional Cardiovascular Medicine (**PCR-EAPCI** textbook). Frederic Doncieux, Veronique Deltort, Paul Cummins, 2012.

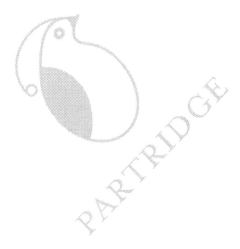

Transseptal Left Heart Catheterisation (TLHC)

Routes for transseptal catheterisation:

1. Right femoral vein. (most common)
2. Left femoral vein. (alternative)
3. Right internal jugular vein. (alternative)

Indications:

1. Severe aortic stenosis: if the valve cannot be crossed, and in patients with aortic prostheses, transseptal catheterisation is done to measure left ventricular pressure and the aortic gradient.
2. To measure the mitral valve gradient in patients with prosthetic mitral valves.
3. To measure the **LVOT** gradient in patients with **HOCM**.
4. Mitral balloon valvuloplasty.
5. Transcatheter mitral valve repair.
6. Left atrial appendage occlusion.
7. Some cases of **PFO** closure.
8. Mitral paravalvular leak closure.
9. Radiofrequency ablation of atrial fibrillation, accessory pathways, and **AV** reentrant tachycardia.

Future indications:

1. Percutaneous mitral valve replacement.
2. Antegrade **TAVI**, through the mitral valve.

Contraindications:

Absolute:

1. Atrial septal thrombus.
2. Atrial septal tumour (myxoma).

Relative:

1. Left atrial body mural thrombus.
2. Left atrial tumors, other than myxoma.
3. Marked enlargement of atria.
4. Prior patch surgical repair of atrial septum or AMPLATZER® Septal Occluder.
5. Severe deformity of the chest or the spine.

Conditions leading to difficulty in performing transseptal puncture:

1. Septum resistant to needle puncture.
2. Bulging septum due to a very high left atrial pressure, causing the needle to slip medially or laterally during the puncture.
3. Giant left atrium, causing difficulty in finding the catch point on the septum.
4. Very large right atrium.
5. Atrial septal aneurysm.

Complications:

1. Air embolism through the catheter.
2. Thromboembolism.
3. Perforation of the aorta.
4. Perforation of the atrial wall leading to haemopericardium.
5. Small **ASD**.

References:

1. Brockenbrough EC, et al. New Technique for Left Ventricular Angiography and Transseptal Left Heart Catheterisation. Am. J. Cardiol. 1960; 6:1062-4

2. Braunwald E. Transseptal Left Heart Catheterisation. Circulation. 1968; 37 (suppl 111): 74-79

3. Clugston R. et al. Transseptal Catheterisation Update 1992. Cathet cardiovasc. Diagnosis. 1992; 26:266-74

4. Hung JS. et al. Atrial Septal Puncture Technique in Percutaneous Mitral Commissurotomy. Cathetcardiovasc. Diagnosis. 1992; 26:275-284

5. Kiwan Y. et al. Mitral Balloon Valvuloplasty. New Emerging Indications. Saudi Heart Journal. Vol 7. No.1, 73-82 August (1995).

6. Shaw TRD. et al. Mitral Balloon Valvotomy and Left Atrial Thrombus. Heart. 2005; 91:1088-1089

7. Percutaneous Interventional Cardiovascular Medicine. (The PCR-EAPCI Textbook). EECKHOUT E. et al. Europa 2012 Edition. Publisher: Frederic Doncieux

Endomyocardial Biopsy (EMB)

Recommendations of EMB:

1. Fulminant unexplained heart failure of duration less than two weeks. (lymphocytic myocarditis, giant cell myocarditis and necrotising eosinophilic myocarditis)

2. Unexplained new onset of heart failure of two to 12-week duration, associated with recent ventricular arrhythmia, **AV** block, or failure to respond to medical treatment. (giant cell myocarditis)

3. Unexplained heart failure, of duration greater than three months, with late arrhythmias, **AV** block or failure to respond to medical treatment. (sarcoidosis, giant cell myocarditis)

4. Unexplained heart failure with dilated cardiomyopathy, of any duration, associated with suspected allergic reaction and eosinophilia. (hypersensitivity myocarditis)

5. Suspected anthracycline cardiotoxicity.

6. In selected patients with heart failure associated with restrictive cardiomyopathy if other workup is inconclusive. (amyloidosis, haemochromatosis)

7. In patients with cardiac tumor if **EMB** is likely to alter the management. (except myxoma)

8. Suspected arrhythmogenic right ventricular cardiomyopathy, if other evaluation tests are inconclusive.

9. Heart failure with unexplained ventricular hypertrophy, if infiltrative or storage diseases (amyloidosis, Fabry's disease) are suspected and other tests are inconclusive.

10. Monitoring cardiac allograft rejection.
11. Acute exacerbation of chronic cardiomyopathy.

Limitations of EMB:

1. It is a safe procedure, but has non-negligible complications.
2. The diagnostic yields of biopsies of both ventricles **(LV** and **RV)** are much more than a biopsy of one ventricle only.
3. Sampling error due to patchy area of inflammation and limitation of the sampling to the subendocardial layers only.

Complications of EMB:

Major complications: (1%)

1. Cardiac tamponade. (0.4%)
2. Pneumopericardium.
3. Complete **AV** block. (0.1%)
4. Stroke.
5. Myocardial infarction.
6. Tricuspid valve regurgitation.
7. Pulmonary or systemic embolisation.
8. Death. (0.03%)

Minor complications: (2-4%)

1. Transient chest pain.
2. Non-sustained **VT**.
3. Transient **AV** block.
4. Transient hypotension

References:

1. Transvenous Right Ventricle Endomyocardial Biopsy in Adult Patients with Cardiomyopathy. J. Am. Coll. Cardiol. 1992; 19:43-7.
2. Deckers J.W. et al. Complications of transvenous right ventricle endomyocardial biopsy in adult patients with cardiomyopathy.J Am Coll Cardiol.1992; 19:43-47.
3. Kiwan Y, Yousuf Ali A., Muscat-Baron J. et al. Endomyocardial Biopsy for Malignant Cardiac Neoplasms: Report of one Case and Review of Literature. Emirates Medical Journal 8,124-127(1997).
4. Ardehali H. et al. Endomyocardial Biopsy Plays a Role in Diagnosing Patients with Unexplained Cardiomyopathy. Am. Heart J. 2004; 147:919-23.
5. Cooper LT. et al. The Role of Endomyocardial Biopsy in the Management of Cardiovascular Diseases. A scientific statement from the AHA. Eu.r Heart J. 2007; 28:3076-93.
6. Leone O. et al. 2011, Consensus Statement on Endomyocardial Biopsy from the Association for European Cardiovascular Pathology and the Society of Cardiovascular Pathology. Cadiovasc. Pathol. 2012; 21-245.

Pericardial Intervention (PI)

Percutaneous Intervention in Pericardial Diseases

1. Percutaneous pericardiocentesis.
2. Percutaneous balloon pericardiotomy.
3. Surgical pericardial window.
4. Intrapericardial injection of sclerosing agents.
5. Percutaneous closed pericardial biopsy.
6. Percutaneous pericardioscopy with biopsy.
7. Percutaneous pericardial access for epicardial mapping and ablation of cardiac arrhythmia

Indications for percutaneous pericardiocentesis: (PPC)

1. Cardiac tamponade or impending tamponade.
2. As a diagnostic approach in effusion of unknown etiology.
3. Infective pericardial effusion where fluid culture is desirable.
4. Recurrent pericardial effusion.
5. Aspiration for palliative reasons.

Contraindications of PPC: (surgical drainage is preferred)

1. Haemopericardium due to aortic dissection, post-myocardial infarction or post-trauma.
2. In patients with bleeding diathesis.
3. Recurrent pericardial effusion.
4. Purulent pericardial effusion.

5. Mild or moderate effusion.
6. Loculated effusion.
7. Posteriorly located effusion.
8. Fungal or tuberculous pericarditis.
9. Chylopericardium for concurrent aspiration of fluid and surgical ligation of the thoracic duct.

Complications of pericardiocentesis:

1. Haemothorax.
2. Perforation of heart leading to cardiac tamponade.
3. Intercostal artery puncture.
4. Coronary artery punctures.
5. Left internal mammary artery puncture.
6. Pleuropericardial fistula.
7. Pneumothorax.
8. Arrhythmias.
9. Perforation of liver, lung.

Management of recurrent pericardial effusion:

1. Percutaneous pericardiocentesis.
2. Percutaneous balloon pericardiotomy.
3. Surgical pericardial window.
4. Intrapericardial injection of sclerosing agents.

Percutaneous closed pericardial biopsy:

Technique first developed by our group in Kuwait in 1988.

1. It is a safe and simple technique which can be performed simultaneously with percutaneous pericardiocentesis.
2. It is a very sensitive diagnostic technique, especially in malignant and tuberculous pericardial effusion.
3. Multiple biopsies from different parts of the parietal pericardium can be obtained.
4. It is performed using fluoroscopic guidance in the catheterisation laboratory.
5. The overall sensitivity is 60%, but is very sensitive in malignant and tuberculous etiology.

Pericardioscopy:

1. Enables direct and percutaneous endoscopic inspection of visceral and parietal pericardium.
2. Enables biopsy of both parietal and visceral pericardium.
3. Is up to 97% sensitivity, and is more sensitive than fluoroscopic closed pericardial biopsy.

Percutaneous balloon pericardiotomy:

1. It is safe and effective alternative to surgical pericardial window.
2. The balloon dilatation of the pericardium allows shifting of pericardial fluid to the pleural or peritoneal space.
3. Usually done with 3.0 cm x 20 mm balloon straddling and dilating the parietal pericardium.

Intrapericardial delivery of sclerosing agents:

1. Tetracycline, doxycycline.
2. Chemotherapeutic agents. (bleomycin, thiotepa)
3. Radioactive phosphorus.

All the above have been used effectively to prevent the recurrence of pericardial effusion.

References:

1. Endrys J, Simo M., Shafie M.Z, Uthman B., Kiwan Y., Chugh T. Ali S.M, Spacek K., Yosuf A.M, Cherian G;A New Non- surgical Technique for Multiple Pericardial Biopsies. Cathet. Cardiovasc. diagn.1988; 15:92-4

2. Palacios IF. et al; Percutaneous Balloon Pericardial Window for Patients With Malignant Pericardial Effusion and Tamponade. Cathet cardiovasc diagn. 1991; 22:244-9

3. Selig MB. et al; Percutaneous Transcatheter Pericardial Intervention : Aspiration, Biopsy and Pericardioplasty. Am. Heart J. 1993; 125:269-71

4. Uthman B. et al; Percutaneous Pericardial BiopsyTechnique, Efficacy, Safety and Value in the Management of Pericardial Effusion. Pediatr cardiol. 1997; 18:414-8

5. Spodick D.H; Acute Cardiac Tamponade. N. Eng. J. Med.2003; 349:684-90

6. Seferovic PM. Et al. Diagnostic Value of Pericardial Biopsy: Improvement with Exclusive Sampling Enabled by Pericardioscopy. Circulation. 2003;107:978-83

Percutaneous Alcohol Septal Ablation (ASA) in Hypertrophic Obstructive Cardiomyopathy

Key points to remember:

1. **ASA** relieves **LVOT** obstruction by creating a localised myocardial infarction in the area of the basal septal muscle where **SAM**-septal contact is occurring. Remodeling of this area of contact leads to widening of the **LVOT**.
2. **ASA** has similar outcome to surgery in terms of improving symptoms, increases exercise capacity improves long-term survival.
3. There are no randomized trials comparing ASA with surgery.
4. Studies have shown that the procedure is safe and effective in most patients.
5. Long-term survival is comparable to historical reports of surgical myectomy and approaches that of the general population.
6. **ASA** is a viable treatment for patients with **HOCM**.
7. **ASA** advantages over surgery include:
   a) Avoidance of surgical sternotomy.
   b) Shorter recovery and shorter hospital stay.
   c) Lower risk of occurrence of **VSD** as a complication.
   d) Treatment of concomitant coronary stenosis by angioplasty.
   e) Less expensive.
   f) Can be repeated.

Causes of left ventricular hypertrophy without obstruction:

1. Hypertrophic non-obstructive cardiomyopathy.
2. Hypertension.
3. Infiltrative heart disease. (amyloidosis, haemochromatosis)
4. Athlete's heart.
5. Drugs (anabolic steroids, tacrolimus, hydroxychloroquin)
6. Malformation syndromes (Noonan).

Common diagnostic challenges in HOCM:

1. Presentation in the late phase of the disease, with dilated and /or hypokinetic left ventricle and wall thinning.
2. Physiological hypertrophy caused by intense athlete training.
3. Patients with co-existent pathologies (hypertension, valvular disease).

Causes of dynamic LVOT obstruction

1. HOCM (common).
2. Calcification of posterior mitral annulus.
3. Hypertension.
4. Hypovolemia.
5. Hypercontractile states.

Causes of syncope in HOCM

1. Hypovolemia
2. Complete heart block
3. Sinus node dysfunction.
4. Ventricular tachycardia.

5. Atrial fibrillation.
6. LVOT obstruction
7. Abnormal vascular reflexes.

Indications of ASA

(IIa B) (ACC/AHA 2011 guidlines)

1. Clinical :
   If the patient is having significant **surgical** comorbidities, **or** there are contraindications to surgery, **or** patients refusing surgery, **with** one or more of the following symptoms:
   a) Symptomatic patients with severe dyspnea
   b) Angina class III, refractory to medical therapy. b) Exercise-induced syncope.

2. Haemodynamic:
   a) Resting gradient > 30 mmHg.
   b) Provoked gradient > 50 mmHg. (by Valsalva manoeuvre, post-extra systole, exercise or drugs)

3. Echocardiographic:
   a) The presence of subaortic gradient with **SAM**. b) Presence of mid-cavity gradient.
   b) Absence of intrinsic mitral valve apparatus disorders.

4. Coronary angiographic:
   The presence of a suitably-sized septal branch artery.

ESC 2014 Guidelines:

1. Septal reduction therapies (myectomy or ASA) have to be performed by experienced operators working as part of a multidisplinary team expert in the management of HOCM. (I A).
2. Septal myectomy rather than ASA is recommended in patients with an indication for septal reduction therapy and other lesions requiring surgical intervention (e.g. Mitral valve repair/replacement, papillary muscle intervention). (I A).

Alcohol septal ablation has:

1. Similar functional improvement to surgical myectomy.
2. A 4-year survival rate similar to surgical myectomy.
3. Ventricular arrhythmias in 5%, which is higher than in surgical myectomy. (0.2%)
4. An uncertain effect in severe septal thickness of above 30 mm.
5. Higher risk of AV block compared to surgery.
6. Higher residual LVOT gradient, than surgery.
7. Higher risk of VSD if septum is 16mm so should be avoided.
8. Is less effective in patients with extensive septal scarring on computed magnetic resonance scan.

Contraindications of ASA:

1. Mild or no symptoms.
2. Hypertrophy not affecting the interventricular septum. (examples include only the apex or the free wall)
3. Absence of intraventricular gradient.
4. Thin septum. (< 16mm)
5. Intrinsic mitral valve abnormalities. (very long and flail leaflets)

6. Anomalous morphology of the papillary muscles insertion.
7. The presence of severe coronary stenoses requiring surgical revascularisation.

Technical considerations:

1. Balloon size average is 1.2 x 6 mm
2. The amount of alcohol is 1 ml for each 1 cm of septum thickness.
3. Select the first big septal branch
4. The septal branches may arise from **LAD**, diagonal, or intermediate arteries.
5. Occasionally you might need to inject into two septal branches.

Signs of success of ablation:

1. 50% reduction of gradient.
2. Decrease in the degree of **SAM**.
3. Decrease in the severity of **MR**.
4. **ST** segment elevation in leads **V1** and **V2**.
5. **ST** segment depression in **V5** and **V6**.
6. **CPK** elevation(>1200).

Complications:

1. Puncture site:
   a) Bleeding and haematoma. b) **AV** fistula.
   b) Femoral pseudoaneurysm.

2. Emergency surgery due to:
   a) Coronary perforation. (very rare)
   b) Severe mitral regurgitation. c) Cardiac tamponade. (1%)

3. Remote extensive myocardial infarction due to:
   a) Coronary dissection. (2%)
   b) Alcohol leakage. (uncommon)

4. Heart blocks:
   a) First degree. (50%)
   b) Right bundle branch block. (50%)
   c) Transient complete heart block. (50%)
   d) Permanent complete heart block. (10%)

5. Ventricular arrhythmias (soon, or late, after ablation), which include ventricular tachycardia and ventricular fibrillation. (2%)

6. Mortality (2% at 30 days and 8% at 5 years) due to:
   a) Left ventricular failure. b) Cardiac tamponade.
   b) Coronary dissection.
   c) Ventricular fibrillation. e) Pulmonary embolism.

Surgical myectomy:

Rarely, the following complications may arise:
   a) Complete heart block. (2%)
   b) **VSD**. (<1%)
   c) Aortic or mitral valve injury. (<1%)
   d) Ventricular arrhythmia. (0.2% per year).

Surgical myectomy / compared to ASA has:

1. Lower incidence of heart block.
2. Lower incidence of ventricular tachycardia.

3. Higher incidence of VSD.

4. Less residual gradient.

References:

1. Alam M. et al. Alcohol Septal Ablation for HOCM, A Systemic Review of Published Studies. J. interv. cardiol. 2006; 19:319.

2. Welge D. et al. Long- term Follow- up after Percutaneous Septal Ablation in HOCM. Dtsch. Med. wochenschr. 2008; 133; 1949-54

3. Rigoploulos A.G. et al. A Decade of Percutaneous Septal Ablation in Hypertrophic Cardiomyopathy. Circ J. 2010; 75:28-37

4. Gersh B.J.et al. 2011 ACCF/AHA Guidelines for the Diagnosis and Treatment of HOCM. JACC. 2011; 13; 124:2761-96

5. Percutaneous Interventional Cardiovascular Medicine. (PCR-EAPCI) Textbook. Frederic Doncieux 2012.

6. 2014 ESC guidelines on the diagnosis and management of hypertrophic cardiomyopathy. European heart journal (2014) 35, 2733-2779.

7. Euro PCR, Paris, may, 2015

Percutaneous Transluminal Coronary Angioplasty (PTCA)

Key Points to Remember:

1. Onsite surgical standby is not mandatory, as emergency surgery is required in only 0.2%.

2. Radial approach is progressing very fast especially during primary PTCA, and in many centers radial is replacing femoral approach and showing lower complications rate.

3. In patients with stable angina not interfering with the quality of life, and when there are no indications of prolonging life (like **LMS** stenting), initial medical therapy, rather than immediate revascularisation, should be tried(except in patients with high risk criteria on noninvasive tests).

4. Certain subsets of LM stenosis are upgraded to class I indication.

5. In patients with NSTEMI, early invasive strategy is recommended over conservative strategy.

6. Optimal timing of angiography for stable patients after successful fibrinolysis is 3-24 hours. (Class IIa A).

7. In patients with diabetes and chronic kidney disease, CABG is still the treatment of choice, rather than PTCA.

8. PTCA of non infarct artery may be considered in selected patients with STEMI and multivessel disease who are hemodynamically stable, either at the time of the primary PTCA or as planned staged procedure, and upgraded to (class IIb B).

9. The usefulness of selective and bailout aspiration thrombectomy in patients undergoing primary PTCA is not well established, and downgraded to. (Class IIb C).

10. Routine aspiration thrombectomy before primary PTCA is not useful, and downgraded to. (Class III A, no benefit).

11. Always remember to be safe physician rather than unsafe technician

Recommendations for revascularisations in patients with stable coronary artery disease:

1. Patients in whom maximum medical therapy did not improve angina symptoms.

2. Patients who are intolerant of medical therapy.

3. Patients with intermediate to high-risk criteria on non- invasive testing, regardless of angina severity.

4. In patients with stable angina not interfering with the quality of life, and when there are no indications of prolonging life (like **LMS** stenting), initial medical therapy, rather than immediate revascularisation, should be tried.

5. After a period of medical therapy, **PTCA** might be considered if patient prefers to avoid future possibility of urgent revascularisation.

Indications of PTCA in patients with stable coronary artery disease:

1. One- or two-vessel disease without proximal **LAD**. (Class I C)

2. One vessel disease with proximal **LAD**. (Class I A)

3. Two-vessel disease with proximal **LAD**. (Class I C)

4. Left main disease with SYNTAX scores ≤ 22. (Class I B)

5. Left main disease with SYNTAX scores 23-32. (Class IIa B)
6. Left main disease with SYNTAX score > 32. (Class III B)
7. Three-vessel disease with SYNTAX scores ≤ 22. (Class I B)
8. Three-vessel disease with SYNTAX score 23-32, or >32. (Class III B).

PTCA in patients with NSTEMI:

1. Urgent coronary angiography (< 2 hours) in patients with a very high ischemic risk (Class I C):
   a) Refractory angina. b) Heart failure.
   b) Cardiogenic shock.
   c) Refractory arrhythmias.
   d) Haemodynamic instability.
2. Early coronary angiogram (< 24 hours) in patients with at least one primary high-risk criterion. (Class I A)
3. Angiogram (< 72 hours) in patients with at least one high- risk criterion. (Class I A)
4. Non-invasive documentation of ischemia is recommended in low-risk patients without recurrent ischemia. (Class I A)

NSTEMI: (high-risk criteria)

- **Primary criteria:**

1. Relevant rise or fall in troponins.
2. Dynamic **ST-T** wave changes.
3. GRACE score > 140.

- **Secondary criteria:**

1. Diabetes mellitus.
2. Renal insufficiency.
3. Ejection fraction < 40%.
4. Recent **PCI**.
5. Prior **CABG**.
6. Intermediate GRACE score.

PTCA: (in STEMI):

1. Primary **PTCA** is recommended over fibrinolysis if performed in a timely fashion within 12 hours of symptom onset. (Class I A)
2. Primary **PTCA** is indicated after 12 hours of onset of chest pain if there is continuing ischemia, arrhythmia or if chest pain and **ECG** changes are stuttering. (Class I C)
3. Primary **PTCA** is indicated for patients with acute heart failure or cardiogenic shock, <u>irrespective</u> of the time of symptoms onset. (Class I B)
4. Primary PTCA should be considered in patients with late presentation (12-48 hours) after symptoms onset. (Class IIa B)
5. **PTCA** of non infarct artery may be considered in selected patients with STEMI and multivessel disease who are hemodynamically stable, either at the time of the primary PTCA or as planned staged procedure (class IIb B).
6. The usefulness of selective and bailout aspiration thrombectomy in patients undergoing primary PTCA is not well established.(IIb C).
7. Routine aspiration thrombectomy before primary PTCA is not useful. (III A, no benefit).

Revascularisation of patients with STEMI (after fibrinolysis):

1. Coronary angiography is recommended within a 24-hour period after successful fibrinolysis. (Class I A)
2. Emergency angiography is indicated in cardiogenic shock or severe heart failure after fibrinolysis. (Class I B) 20
3. Emergency rescue **PTCA** is indicated when fibrinolysis has failed at 60 minutes (< 50% ST resolution or persistent chest pain). (Class I A)
4. Emergency **PTCA** is indicated for recurrent ischemia, haemodynamic instability, and threatening ventricular arrhythmias after initial successful fibrinolysis. (Class I A)
5. Optimal timing of angiography for stable patients after successful fibrinolysis is 3-24 hours. (Class IIa A)

PTCA: (in patients with chronic kidney disease)

1. **CABG** should be considered over **PTCA** in patients with multi-vessel **CAD**, with acceptable surgical risk. (Class IIa B)
2. In patients with high surgical risk, **PTCA** should be considered. (Class IIa B)

PTCA: (in patients with diabetes)

1. In patients with **STEMI**, primary **PTCA** is recommended over fibrinolysis. (Class I A)
2. In patients with **N-STEMI**, an early invasive strategy is recommended over non-invasive strategy. (Class I A)
3. In patients with stable multi-vessel **CAD, CABG** is recommended over **PTCA**. (Class I A)

4. In patients with stable multi-vessel **CAD** and SYNTAX score ≥ 22, PTCA should be considered as an alternative to **CABG**. (Class IIa B)

Complications of coronary angioplasty:

1. Vascular access complications. (1%)
2. Retroperitoneal bleeding. (0.2%)
3. Renal failure. (0.3%)
4. Stent thrombosis. (1-2%)
5. Emergency surgery. (0.2%)
6. Myocardial infarction. (0.2%)
7. Cardiac perforation. (0.3%)
8. Stroke. (0.3%)
9. Death in catheterisation laboratory. (0.05%)

Local complications of transfemoral access:

1. Femoral artery dissection.
2. Femoral **AV** fistula.
3. Pseudoaneurysm.
4. Haematoma.
5. Retroperitoneal haemorrhage.
6. Femoral artery thrombosis.
7. Infection.

Local complications of transradial access:

1. Radial dissection.
2. Radial vasospasm.
3. Radial perforation with haematoma.

4. Pseudoaneurysm.
5. Compartment syndrome.
6. Switching rate to femoral approach is 5%.
7. Radial occlusion is 5%.
8. The surgeon cannot use the radial artery for future grafting.

Indications for emergency surgery in PTCA:

1. Aortic dissection.
2. Coronary perforation with tamponade.
3. Extensive coronary dissection.
4. Guide wire fracture.
5. Haemodynamic instability.

Golden rules to avoid complications in PTCA:

1. Know your own limitations (be safe physician, not unsafe technician).
2. Proper patient and lesion selection.
3. Avoid oculostenotic reflex.
4. Selection of proper equipment.
5. Keep the procedure as simple as possible.
6. Know when to stop, and ask for help if needed.
7. Maintain the highest levels of concentration.
8. Learn from your own, and others' mistakes.
9. Always update yourself with the latest international guidelines.

References:

1. Klein L.W., Coronary Complications of Percutaneous Coronary Intervention. Catheter. Cardiovasc Interven. 2005; 64-395-401

2. Silber S. et al. Guidelines for Percutaneous Coronary Interventions. Eur. E. J. 2005; 26:804-47

3. Percutaneous Interventional Cardiovascular Medicine (The PCR-EAPCI Textbook). Frederic Doncieux, Veronique Deltort, Paul Cummins, 2012.

4. Windecker S. 2014 ESC/EACTS Guidelines on Myocardial Revascularisation. European Heart Journal. Online, 30 August 2014.

5. Levine GN, et al.2015 ACC/AHA/SCAI Focused Update on Primary PCI, online, October 2015, doi;10.1002/ccd.26325

Mitral Balloon Valvuloplasty (MBV)

Key points to remember:

1. Symptomatic patients with severe MS(MVA <1.5cm2) always need dilatation.
2. However Asymptomatic patients with severe MS can also be dilated if they have high risk criteria (previous embolisation, PAF, Pulmonary hypertension, a desire for pregnancy).
3. Unfavorable criteria are old age, close mitral commissurotomy, AF, Severe pulmonary hypertension, and high Wilkins score of > 8.
4. There are only two absolute contra indications (fresh mobile LA body thrombus and MS without fusion of commissures).
5. The existing **MR** can either increase or decrease or remain the same after dilatation.
6. The interatrial shunt is usually small and has no consequences and usually closes spontaneously.
7. Dilation of coexisting aortic and tricuspid valve stenoses can be done in the same sitting.

Indications:

Severe MS (MVA < 1.5cm²)

1. <u>Symptomatic</u> patients with favorable valve morphology in the absence of left atrial thrombus or moderate-severe **MR**. (Class IA)
2. <u>Symptomatic</u> patients with suboptimal valve pathology, and either contraindications to, or high risk for surgery. (Class IIb C)

3. <u>Symptomatic</u> patients with unfavorable anatomy but favorable clinical characteristics. (Class IIa C)
4. <u>Asymptomatic</u> patients with favorable morphology and very severe **MS** (**MVA** < 1 cm²). (Class IIa C)
5. <u>Asymptomatic</u> patients with severe **MS** < 1.5cm² and having one of the following : (6 p)
   a) Previous history of embolism.
   b) Dense spontaneous echo contrast in left atrium.
   c) Paroxysmal atrial fibrillation.
   d) Pulmonary hypertension. (> 50 mmHg)
   e) Patients in need of major non-cardiac surgery.
   f) A desire for pregnancy.

Unfavorable clinical characteristics:

1. Old age.
2. Previous close mitral commissurotomy.
3. Atrial fibrillation.
4. Severe pulmonary artery hypertension.

Unfavorable anatomic characteristics:
Wilkins score > 8.

Contraindications:

1. Fresh mobile left atrial thrombus. (Absolute)
2. Mitral regurgitation. (more than moderate)
3. Severe commissural calcifications.
4. Mitral stenosis without fusion of commissures. (Absolute)

5. Association of severe aortic valve disease or coronary artery disease. (Relative)
6. Mitral valve area of > 1.5 cm2.

Author's experience:

Mitral balloon valvuloplasty **can** be performed in the following situations:

1. **Organized** left atrial mural thrombus.
2. Intracavity, non-protruding, non-mobile left atrial **Appendage** thrombus.
3. **Bi-commissural** calcification.
4. **Associated** severe rheumatic non-calcified **aortic** valve stenosis or tricuspid valve stenosis, where mitral, aortic, and **tricuspid** valve dilatations can be performed in the same sitting.

Complications:

1. Embolism (0.5-5%)
   due to:
   a) Thrombus in left atrium. b) Thrombus in catheter.
   b) Air leaking from balloon. d) Calcium.

2. Haemopericardium (0.5 - 8%) Due to:
   a) Perforation by Transseptal needle.
   b) Perforation by Guide wires.
   c) Perforation by Balloons. (Inoue balloon has the least complications)

3. Severe mitral regurgitation (2%-12%) Due to:
   a) Leaflets tearing
   b) Rupture chordae
   c) Rupture of papillary muscle
   d) Excessive commissural splitting

4. Inter-atrial shunt. (10-90%)
   In the **AUTHOR's** experience: The shunt is:
   a) Usually small, and have no consequences.
   b) Least shunt is with Inoue balloon.
   c) Usually close spontaneously within few months.
   d) Very rarely, surgical closure is required.

5. Arrhythmias.
   a) Atrial fibrillation. (rare)
   b) Transient complete heart block. (< 1%)
   c) Bacterial endocarditis. (very rare)

6. Mortality. (0%-3%) Due to:
   a) Massive haemopericardium or
   b) Patient comorbidities.

References:

1. Inoue K. et al. Clinical Application of Transvenous Mitral Comissurotomy by a New Balloon Catheter. J. thorac cardiovasc surg. 1984; 87:394-402.
2. Gharbo H, Vijay V., Endrys J., Kiwan Y. Incidence of ASD Following Percutaneous Mitral Balloon Valvuloplasty (abstract). The 1st Pan-Arab Congress of Cardiology and the 17th Annual Meeting of the Egyptian Society of Cardiology. Cairo, Egypt, Feb. 1990.

3. Kiwan Y. et al. Combined Percutaneous Aortic and Mitral Balloon Valvuloplasty in Patients with Severe Rrheumatic Aortic and Mitral Stenosis. Journal of Saudi Heart Association, vol 3, No.2. 1991.

4. Iung B. et al. Usefulness of Percutaneous Balloon Comissurotomy for Mitral Stenosis During Pregnancy. Am. J. cardiol. 1994; 73:398-400.

5. Vahanian A. et al. Percutaneous Transvenous Mitral Commissurotomy Using Inoue Balloon: cathet. cardiovasc Diagn. 1994; 2:8-15.

6. Kiwan Y. et al., Mitral Balloon Valvuloplasty by Inoue Technique without Echocardiographic Standby. Annals of Saudi medicine. 1994, 14(5): 375-378.

7. Kiwan Y. et al. Mitral Balloon Valvuloplasty: New Emerging Indications. Saudi Heart Journal. Vol 7. No. 1, 73-82. August 1995.

8. Complications and Mortality of Percutaneous Balloon Mitral Commissurotomy. Am. J. Cardiol. 2002; 90:1170-73.

9. Gamra H. et al. Balloon Mitral Commissurotomy in Juvenile Rheumatic Mitral Stenosis. A ten-year clinical and Echocardiographic Actuarial Results. Eur. Heart J. 2003; 24:11349-56.

10. ESC 2012, Guidelines on the Management of Valvular Heart Disease. Vahanian A. et al. European Heart Journal. Online: 25 August 2012.

11. ACC/AHA 2014 Guidelines for the Management of Valvular Heart Disease. Nishimura R. A. et al. Circulation. 2014, 129.

Pulmonary Balloon Valvuloplasty (PBV)

Indications:

(Balloon valvuloplasty is the treatment of choice for patient with sever pulmonary stenosis)

1. If echocardiographic transvalvular peak gradient is > 64 mmHg irrespective of symptoms. (invasive gradient > 40 mmHg) (Class I C)
2. Valvuloplasty should be considered with a gradient < 64 mmHg (Class IIa C) in the presence of:
   a) Symptoms related to valvular pulmonary stenosis, or b) Impaired right ventricle function, or
   b) Arrhythmias, or
   c) Right to left intracardiac shunt through **ASD** or **VSD**.

Complications:

Major complications:

1. Rupture of right ventricle outflow tract leading to cardiac tamponade.
2. Injury to tricuspid valve with resulting significant tricuspid regurgitation.
3. Moderate or severe pulmonary regurgitation.

Minor complications:

1. Transient arrhythmias.
2. Femoral vein thrombosis.
3. Dynamic infundibular obstruction resulting in hypotension.

References:

1. Nugent E.W. et al. Clinical Course in Pulmonary Stenosis. Circulation. 1977; 56:138-47
2. Fawzy M.E. et al. Late Results of Pulmonary Balloon Valvuloplasty in Adults Using Double Balloon Technique. J. intervent cardiol. 1988; 1:35-42
3. Mendelson A.M. et al. Predictors of Successful Pulmonary Balloon Valvuloplasty: 10- year experience. Cathet. Cardiovasc Diagn. 1996; 39:236
4. Baumgartner H. et al. 2010 ESC Guidelines for the Management of Grown-up Congenital Heart Disease. Eur. Heart J. 2010.

Aortic Balloon Valvuloplasty (ABV)

Indications:

1. In selected adolescent and young adults with non- calcified valve balloon valvuloplasty may be considered.
2. In calcific aortic stenosis: might be considered as a bridge to surgery or **TAVI**. (Class IIb C)
3. As a routine procedure prior to **TAVI**.
4. ABV is considered as the first-line therapy in congenital aortic stenosis.

Complications:

1. Vascular. (4-12%)
2. Stroke. (1-3%)
3. Annular rupture. (0.3%)
4. Cardiac tamponade.
5. Severe aortic regurgitation. (1-2%)
6. Mortality. (4-10%)

References:

1. Cribrier A. et al. Percutaneous Transluminal Valvuloplasty of Acquired Aortic Stenosis in Elderly Patients: An Alternative to Valve Replacement? Lancet. 1986; 63-7

2. Letac B. et al. Results of Percutenous Transluminal Valvuloplasty in 218 Patients with Valvular Aortic Stenosis. Am. J. Cardiol. 1988; 598-605

3. NHLBI Balloon Valvuloplasty Registry. Circulation. 1991; 84:2383-97

4. Kiwan Y. et al. Combined Percutaneous Aortic and Mitral Balloon Valvuloplasty in Patients with Severe Rheumatic Aortic and Mitral Stenosis. Journal of Saudi Heart Association. Vol 3, No.2. 1991.

5. Kiwan Y. et al. Balloon Dilatation for Discrete Subaoric Membraneous Stenosis, Immediate and Short Term Results.Saudi Heart Journal, vol. 5, No, 1, may 1994.

6. Baumgartner H. et al. 2010 ESC Guidelines for the Management of Grown-up Congenital Heart Disease. Eur. Heart J. 2010.

7. ACC/AHA 2014 Guidelines for the Management of Valvular Heart Disease. Nishimura R.A. et al. Circulation. 2014; 129.

Transcatheter Aortic Valve Implantation (TAVI)

Key points to remember:

1. Surgical AVR remains the treatment of choice for symptomatic severe aortic stenosis.
2. The current guidelines indications are only in patients with high or prohibitive risks for surgery.
3. Uptill now we do not have any solid data telling us when to intervene in patients who are not bothered by their AS (asymptomatic).
4. AR is common and is linked with increased mortality.
5. There is high incidence of conduction disturbances and pace maker insertion.
6. Stroke rate is about 7%, however silent cerebral infarcts by MRI are seen in about 70% of patients.
7. TAVI is progressing fast and valve in valve TAVI is getting popularity.
8. 70% of patients developed silent myocardial damage, manifested by increase in the level of CPK, this is linked with higher mortality in this group of patients.

Severity of Aortic Stenosis (by Echocardiography)

Severe AS

1. Aortic velocity ≥ 4 m/s.
2. Mean aortic gradient ≥ 40 mmHg.

3. Peak aortic gradient ≥ 60 mmHg.
4. AVA ≤ 1.0 cm².

Very severe AS

1. Velocity ≥ 5 m/s.
2. Mean gradient ≥ 50 mmHg.
3. Peak gradient >100 mmHg.

Symptoms of AS

1. Exertional dyspnea.
2. Decreased exercise tolerance.
3. Exertional angina.
4. Presyncope or syncope.

Summary of recommendations of aortic valve replacement; (By either surgical or transcatheter approach)

1. Symptomatic severe **AS**. (Class I B)
2. Asymptomatic severe **AS** and **LVEF** < 50%. (Class I B)
3. Symptomatic patient with low-flow or low gradient severe **AS** with reduced **LVEF** (< 50%) and **AVA** < 1.0cm² and velocity < 4 m/s and mean gradient < 40 mmHg, with increasing velocity and gradient (> 4 m/s and 40 mmHg) during dobutamine test. (Class IIa B)
4. Very severe **AS** (asymptomatic) and a low surgical risk. (Class IIA B)
5. Asymptomatic, severe **AS** with reduced exercise tolerance during exercise treadmill test. (Class IIa B)

Indications of TAVI:

1. **TAVI** is recommended in patients who meet the indications criteria for **AVR** and who are having prohibitive risks for surgical **AVR** and predicted survival greater than 12 months. (Class IB)
2. **TAVI** is a reasonable alternative to surgical **AVR** in patients who meet the indications for **AVR** and who have high surgical risk for surgical **AVR**. (Class IIa B)
3. Percutaneous aortic balloon dilatation may be considered as bridge to surgical **AVR** or **TAVI**. (Class IIb C)
4. **TAVI** is not recommended for patients who have comorbidities that would make the expected benefit of correction of aortic stenosis unnecessary. (Class III) (no benefit)

Prohibitive risks for surgery

1. Predicted risk with surgery, of death or major morbidity of > 50% at 1 year, or
2. > 3 major organ system compromise, or
3. Severe procedure-specific impediments.

High risks for surgery

1. **STS** risk estimate > 8%, or
2. Moderate to severe frailty, or
3. 2 major organ system compromise, or
4. Possible procedure-specific impediments.

Major organ system compromise:

1. Severe **LV** dysfunction.
2. Fixed pulmonary hypertension.

3. **CKD** stage 3 or more.
4. Pulmonary dysfunction.
5. Gastrointestinal and liver dysfunction.
6. Cancer.

Procedure-specific impediments for surgery

1. Presence of tracheotomy.
2. Heavily calcified ascending aorta.
3. Chest malformation.
4. Radiation damage.

Contraindications of TAVI

1. Severe organic mitral regurgitation.
2. Bicuspid aortic valve.
3. Aneurysm of ascending aorta.
4. Left ventricle thrombus.
5. Severe coronary disease not amenable to angioplasty.

Complications of TAVI:

Cardiac complications:

1. Coronary ostial occlusion and myocardial infarction (1%)

2. Aortic regurgitation. (common, valvular and paravalvular)
   a) Mild is very common. (70%)
   b) Moderate to severe. (11%)

Causes of aortic regurgitation

a) Valve under-sizing. b) Valve malposition.

b) Valve malapposition.

c) Severe aortic calcification. e) Large annulus diameter.

3. Conduction disturbance. a) **LBBB**. (30%-60%)

    a) Second-degree heart block.

    b) Third-degree heart block (4-21%) depending on type of valve.

    c) Pace maker needed in (14%)

4. Cardiac arrhythmias:

    a) Atrial fibrillation. (6%)

    b) Ventricular tachycardia and fibrillation. (4%-21%)

5. Cardiac perforation with cardiac tamponade. (3%-4%)

6. Aortic root rupture. (< 1%)

7. Prosthetic valve dysfunction leading to valvular stenosis, valvular regurgitation or a combination of both.

8. Valve embolisation (very rare) either during or after procedure.

9. Valve thrombosis (very rare)

10. Endocarditis (rare)

11. Mitral valve injury (very rare)

12. All-cause mortality (7%)

13. 70% of patients developed silent myocardial damage, manifested by increase in the level of CPK, this is linked with higher mortality in this group of patients.

Non-cardiac complications:

1. Stroke. (7%)
   (**However**, silent cerebral infarcts by **MRI** are seen in 70% of patients.)

2. Vascular access injury. (2-30%)
   a) Dissection.
   b) Rupture.
   c) Thrombosis.
   d) **AV** fistula.
   e) Pseudoaneurysms.

3. Acute renal failure (5%)

References:

1. Webb JG. et al. TAVI: Impact on Clinical and Valve-Related Outcomes. Circulation. 2009; 119:3009-16
2. Leon M.B. et al. Transcatheter Aortic Valve Implantation for Aortic Stenosis in Patients Who Cannot Undergo Surgery. N. Eng. J. Med. 2010; 363:1597-607
3. Rodes-cabau J. et al. Transcatheter Aortic Valve Implantation for the Treatment of Severe Aortic Stenosis in Patients with Very High or Prohibitive Surgical Risk. J. Am. Coll. Cardiol. 2010; 55:1080-90
4. ACC/AHA 2014 Guidelines for the Management of Valvular Heart Disease. Nishimura R.A. et al. Circulation. 2014; 129.
5. Euro PCR, Paris, may,2015

Transcatheter Mitral Valve Interventions

There are 2 types of interventions:

1. Transcatheter mitral valve **repair** (**TMVR**): more on that below.
2. Transcatheter mitral valve **replacement:** a procedure in which the valve is inserted either through:
   a) The transapical left ventricular route, or
   b) Through the transseptal route.

Note: A reported thirty patients have been implanted successfully with dedicated mitral valves.

Transcatheter mitral valve repair (TMVR):

Types of TMVR:

1. **Indirect** mitral annuloplasty:
   Which is the placement of a mitral annuloplasty ring to reduce the annular circumference of the mitral valve by placing the device, through the coronary sinus, into the mitral annulus?
   a) It is the simplest and least invasive approach.
   b) Its main limitations are the indirect relationship of the coronary sinus to the mitral annulus.
   c) There is a potential risk of coronary artery compression.

d) Early clinical results have demonstrated the reduction of MR, and clinical benefits.

e) Further trials of the device are ongoing.

2. Direct mitral annuloplasty with the Mitralign® ring: Using the direct aortic route for access to the left ventricle, the device is implanted directly into the sub annular space and the device is anchored to the mitral annulus with two pairs of wires. Clinical trials are ongoing.

3. Percutaneous mitral leaflet repair with the **Mitra Clip®** device: The clip is Dacron–covered and will engage the anterior and posterior mitral leaflets to maintain coaptation.

   a) Clinical improvement of the patient is comparable to conventional mitral surgery.

   b) The reduction of the **MR** grade is not as good as in surgery.

   c) Safer than surgery.

Transcatheter Mitral Valve Repair (TMVR)

Indications:

1. Transcatheter mitral valve repair may be considered for severely symptomatic patients with chronic severe **primary MR**, who have **favorable** anatomy for the repair procedure, and a reasonable life expectancy, and having prohibitive surgical risk due to severe comorbidities. (Class IIa B).

2. **Observational** studies suggest that **TMVR** using a Mitra Clip can reduce mitral regurgitation and improve symptoms in patients with **secondary** (functional) **MR**.

Contraindications:

1. Rheumatic mitral valve disease.
2. Active endocarditis of mitral valve.
3. Intracardiac thrombus.

Echocardiographic criteria for TMVR:

1. Minimum leaflet calcification in the grasping area.
2. Mitral valve area by planimetry is > 4 cm^2.
3. The jet area of MR is > 6cm^2 or $> 30\%$ of left atrial area.

Complications: (overall 17%)

1. Access site bleeding. (13%)
2. Clip embolisation. (very rare)
3. Partial clip detachment. (3%)
4. Mitral stenosis. (0.8%)
5. Infective endocarditis. (very rare)

References:

1. Franzen O. et al. Acute Outcomes of Mitral clip Therapy for Mitral Regurgitation in High-surgical-risk Patients: Emphasis on Adverse Valve Morphology and Severe L.V dysfunction. Eur. Heart J. 2010; 31:1373-81
2. Feldman T. et al. (EVEREST II trial). Percutaneous Repair or Surgery for Mitral Regurgitation. N. Eng. J. Med.2011; 364:1395-406
3. Pleger S.T. et al. Acute Safety and 30-day Outcome After Percutaneous Edge-to-Edge Repair of Mitral Regurgitation in Very High-risk Patients. Am. J. Cardiol. 2011; 108:1478-82

4. Feldman T. et al. Percutaneous Approach to Valve Repair for Mitral Regurgitation. JACC 2014; 63:2057

5. ACC/AHA 2014 Guidelines for the Management of Valvular Heart Disease. Nishimura R.A. et al. Circulation.2014, 129

6. Euro PCR, Paris, may,2015

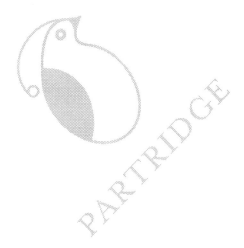

Percutaneous Closure of Paravalvular Leaks (PCPVL)

Key points to remember:

1. Can be asymptomatic.

2. Can cause volume overload with symptoms of heart failure.

3. Can cause severe haemolysis as a result of sheer stress on the red blood cells passing through the leak.

4. Is a common complication of valve replacement. (15% of **MVR**, 10% of **AVR**)

5. Surgical repair is considered the treatment of choice.

6. **PCPVL** is an attractive alternative to surgery, especially in patients considered as high-risk for surgery.

7. Some results of PCPVL showed superiority over surgical repair with a lower complication rate.

8. The following three approaches are available:
   a) Transseptal puncture.
   b) Retrograde transaortic.
   c) Direct transapical left ventricle puncture.

9. Three-dimensional **TOE** provides an accurate assessment of the location and dimensions of the leak prior to, during, and after the procedure.

10. Current **ACC/AHA** 2014 guidelines recommend percutaneous repair of paravalvular regurgitation is reasonable in patients with a prosthetic heart valve who **have**: (Class IIa B)
    a) intractable haemolysis,
    b) severe heart failure,
    c) are considered high-risk for surgery,
    d) anatomical features suitable for catheter-based therapy,
    e) The procedure performed in centers with expertise in the procedure.

Clinical outcomes:

1. Procedural success rate is variable (from 65-90%), depending on the anatomical location of the leak.
2. Haemolysis may not resolve, and may continue until the device is endothelised, after a few months.
3. Symptoms of heart failure usually improve after a few weeks.
4. A second procedure might be needed for a residual paravalvular leak with haemolysis.

Causes of procedural failure:

1. Device interference with the function of the prosthetic valve.
2. Instability of the device with the risk of device embolisation.
3. Inability to cross the paravalvular defect with the guide wire or with the delivery sheath.

Contraindications:

1. Intracardiac thrombi.
2. Severe transvalvular regurgitation.

Complications:

1. Local access site:
   a) Bleeding.
   b) Vessel dissection.
   c) Pseudoaneurysm.
   d) AV fistula.

2. Complications of transseptal puncture:
   a) Cardiac tamponade.
   b) Conduction abnormalities.

3. Device-related complications:
   a) Device embolisation.
   b) Device causing erosion.
   c) Device interference with prosthetic valve function.
   d) Coronary ostial occlusion by the device.

4. Other complications:
   a) Stroke.
   b) Endocarditis.
   c) Development of new haemolysis.
   d) Mortality (4.6% - 20%) depending on the duration of the follow-up.

References:

1. De Almeida Branduo C.M. et al; Multivariate Analysis of Risk Factors for Hospital Mortality in Valvular Reoperations for Prosthetic Valve Dysfunction. Eur. J. Cardiothorac surg. 2002; 22:922-6

2. Hein et al; Catheter Closure of Paravalvular Leak. Eurointervention. 2006; 2:318-25

3. Exposito V. et al; Repeat Mitral Valve Replacement: 30- year Experience. Rev. Esp. Cardiol. 2009; 62; 929-32

4. Sorajja P.et al; Percutaneous Repair of Paravalvular Prosthetic Regurgitation. Circcardiovasc Interv. 2011; 4:314-21

5. Ruiz C.E. et al; Clinical Outcomes in Patients Undergoing Percutaneous Closure of Periprosthetic Paravalvular Leak. J. Am. Coll. Cardiol. 2011; 58:2210-17

6. Jelnin V. et al; Clinical Experience with Percutaneous Left Ventricular Transapical Access for Interventions in Structural Heart Defects; a Safe Access and Secure Exit. JACC cardiovasc interv. 2011:4; 868-74

7. Nishimura R.A. et alACC/AHA 2014, Guidelines for the Management of Valvular Heart Disease. Circulation.2014; 129.

Percutaneous Closure of Atrial Septal Defect

Types of atrial septal defect (ASD):

1. Secundum. (80%)
2. Primum. (15%)
3. Superior sinus venosus defect. (5%)
4. Inferior sinus venosus defect. (1%)
5. Coronary sinus defect. (1%)

Key points to remember:

1. The presence of significant **ASD** usually warrants intervention regardless of symptoms.
2. Closure of **ASD** leads to regression of symptoms, **RV** size, and pulmonary pressure.
3. The success rate of closure is 96%.
4. Low complication rate of <0.5%.
5. 80% of secundum **ASD** are amenable to percutaneous closure.
6. ASD's larger than 38 mm are better treated with surgery.
7. 5% of secundum **ASD**'s show multiple defects which may require multiple devices.
8. Catheter closure has a comparable success rate but lower mortality rates and is more cost effective than surgery.
9. Dual antiplatelet therapy should continue for six months after device closure.

10. Endocarditis prophylaxis is recommended for duration of six months after device closure.

Indications for percutaneous closure

1. Patients with significant shunt (Qp/Qs >1.5 /1) and pulmonary vascular resistance < 5 wood units and signs of **RV** volume overload should undergo **ASD** closure regardless of symptoms. (Class IB)
2. Device closure is the method of choice when applicable. (Class IC)
3. All **ASD**'s should be considered for intervention if there is suspicion of paradoxical embolisation, regardless of size. (IIa C)
4. Closure must be avoided in patients with Eisenmenger physiology. (Class III)

Surgical closure is indicated in

the following cases:

1. Large **ASD**. (> 38 mm in diameter)
2. Absent rims in more than 2 areas.
3. Device is too large to fit in the atria.
4. Sinus venosus and coronary sinus defects.
5. Presence of associated anomalous pulmonary venous drainage.

Complications:

In general, complications are low (1%)

1. Air or clot embolisation.
2. Device embolisation, to the right and left hearts. (early and late)

3. Thrombi on the device, with the risk of stroke.
4. Cardiac perforation, early and late, due to erosion of atrial wall or the aorta. (0.07%)
5. Aortic insufficiency
6. Mitral insufficiency
7. Pulmonary vein thrombosis
8. Endocarditis. (very rare)

References:

1. Roos-hesselink J.W. et al. Excellent Survival and Low Incidence of Arrhythmias, Stroke and Heart Failure; long- term after- surgical ASD Closure at Young Age. A Prospective Follow- up, A Study of 21-23 Years. Eur. Heart J. 2003; 24:1907
2. Webb G. et al. Atrial Septal Defect in the Adult: Recent Progress and Overview. Circulation. 2006; 114:1645-53
3. Baumgartner H. et al. E.S.C.Guidelines for the Management of Grown-up Congenital Heart Disease. Eur. Heart J. 2010; 31:2915-57
4. Majunk N. et al. Closure of ASD with AMPLATZER® Septal Occluder in Adults. Am. J. Cardiol. 2009; 103:550-4
5. Humenberger M. et al., Benefit of Atrial Septal Defect Closure in Adults: Impact of Age. Eur. Heart J. 2011; 32:553-60

Percutaneous Closure of Patent Foramen Ovale (PFO)

Key points to remember:

1. There are many case reports of large thrombus hanging at the **PFO**, detected by echocardiography.

2. The presence of **PFO** with or without septal aneurysm is of uncertain importance for the development of a first or recurrent stroke.

3. It is possible that closure of the **PFO** will:
   a) Reduce the risk of recurrent cryptogenic ischemic stroke.
   b) Reduce migrainous attacks.
   c) Somewhat reduce decompression illness in divers. d) Reduce recurrence of systemic embolisation.

4. Meta-analysis of seven major randomised trials including CLOSURE I, **PC** and RESPECT showed that **PFO** closure did not offer significant benefit over medical therapy for the prevention of recurrent ischemic stroke.

5. Several national registries and observational studies (non-randomised) have shown significant benefit of device closure of **PFO** over medical therapy for the prevention of recurrence of stroke.

6. Additional randomised trials are still needed to decide whether **PFO** closure is superior to medical therapy.

7. The 2014 **AHA/ASA** guidelines for the prevention of stroke conclude that the available body of data does not support a benefit of **PFO** closure for patients with cryptogenic stroke without evidence of **DVT**. If DVT is present, then PFO closure might be considered. (Class IIb C).

8. However, extended 10 years follow-up of the RESPECT trial (presented in TCT October 2015), those patients who had cryptogenic stroke for intention to treat population, patients with **PFO** closure had 54% relative risk reduction for recurrent cryptogenic stroke compared to patients treated with anticoagulant therapy.

Clinical manifestations of PFO:

a) Most patients with **PFO** remain asymptomatic.
b) Potential manifestations and associations are with:

    1. Cryptogenic stroke.
    2. Systemic embolisation.
    3. Migraine and vascular headaches.
    4. Decompression sickness.
    5. Air embolism.
    6. Platypnea – orthodeoxia syndrome. (Dyspnea and desaturation in upright position).
    7. Coronary embolisation with resultant myocardial infarction.

References:

1. Torti S.R. et al. Risk of Decompression Illness Among 230 Divers in Relation to the Presence and Size of Patent Foramen Ovale. Eur. Heart J. 2004; 25:1014-20
2. Alleman Y. et al. Patent Foramen Ovale and High Altitude Pulmonary Edema, J. AM.A 2006; 296:2954-8
3. Whorle J. et al. Closure of Patent Foramen Ovale after Cryptogenic Stroke. Lancet. 2006; 368:350-2
4. Dowson A. et al; (MIST) Tiral to Evaluate the Effectiveness of PFO Closure to Resolve Refractory Migraine Headaches. Circulation. 2008; 117:1397-404
5. Johansson M.C. et al. The Significance of Patent Foramen Ovale. A Current Review of Associated Conditions andTreatment. Int. J. Cardiol. 2009;13; 17-24
6. Kearney L.G. et al; Thrombus Entrapped in a Patent Foramen Ovale. Heart lung. Circ. 2010; 19:58-60
7. Furlan A.J. et al; Closure I Trial. N Eng. J. Med. 2012; 366:991-9
8. Kernan W. et al; The 2014 AHA/ASA Guidelines for the Prevention of Stroke in Patients with Stroke and TIA, Stroke, July 2014; 45
9. TCT San Francisco, October 2015

Percutaneous Closure of Ventricular Septal Defect (VSD)

Types of VSD:

1. Perimembranous (80%), adjacent to aortic and tricuspid valve.
2. Muscular (15%), spontaneous closure is frequent.
3. Outlet (< 5%), often associated with progressive aortic regurgitation.
4. Inlet (**AV** canal type) (1%), seen in Down's syndrome.

Complications of untreated VSD with advancing age:

1. Endocarditis. (0.2%)
2. Heart failure.
3. Discrete subaortic stenosis. (rare)
4. In outlet **VSD**, a prolapse of aortic cusp can cause progressive aortic regurgitation.
5. Arrhythmias.
6. Complete heart block.(rare)

Surgical/Catheter interventional treatments:

- **Surgical** closure remains the treatment of choice. (Mortality 1-2%)
- **Trans-catheter** closure can be considered in:

1. Patients with increased risk factors for surgery.
2. Multiple previous cardiac surgical interventions.

3. In **VSD's** which are poorly accessible for surgical closure.
4. In centrally-located muscular **VSD's**, it can be considered as an alternative to surgery.
5. It has been shown that it is feasible in perimembranous **VSD's**.
6. Can be considered as the treatment of first choice in residual post-surgical **VSD**.
7. 2-4 weeks after post-myocardial infarctions, catheter closure can be considered as the first treatment of choice

Complications of device closure: (98% success rate)

1. Embolisation of the device. (2%)
2. Aortic regurgitation. (3%)
3. Tricuspid regurgitation. (2%)
4. Conduction disturbances with complete heart block. (2%)
5. Transient haemolysis. (2%)
6. Cardiac perforation. (0.5%)

References:

1. Szkutnik M. et al. Post- Infarction V.S.D. Closure with AMPLATZER® Occluder. Eur. J. cardio-thorac surg. 2003; 23:323-7.
2. Roos-Hesselink J.W. et al. Outcome of Patients after Surgical Closure of V.S.D. at Young Age. Eur. Heart J. 2004; 25: 1057-62.
3. Thanopoulos B.D. et al. Outcome of Transcatheter Closure of Muscular V.S.D. with AMPLATZER® Occluder. Heart. 2005; 91:513-6.
4. Butera G. et al. Transcatheter Closure of Perimembranous V.S.D.: Early and Long-term Results. J. Am. Coll. Cardiol. 2007; 50:1189.
5. Caminati M. et al. Transcatheter Closure of Congenital V.S.D: Results of European Registry. Eur. Heart J. 2007; 28:2361.

6. Baumgartner H. et al. ESC Guidelines for the Management of Grown- up Congenital Heart Disease. Eur. Heart J. 2010; 31:2915-57.

7. Zuo J. et al. Results of Transcatheter Closure of Perimembranous V.S.D. Am. J. Cardiol. 2010; 106:1034-7.

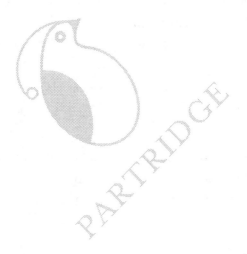

Left Atrial Appendage Occlusion (LAAO)

Key points to remember:

1. 90% of thrombi originate in **LAA** and 10% in other regions of the left atrium. (There might be a need for anticoagulation even after removal or closure of **LAA**)
2. Not all strokes in **AF** patients are cardio-embolic or are due to the AF itself.
3. Inconsistent results of surgical excision or occlusion of **LAA**.
4. Several studies have shown the feasibility of percutaneous **LAA** occlusion.
5. At present, the percutaneous closure is not considered simply as an alternative to anticoagulant therapy.
6. The current recommendations are based mainly on observational studies and registries only.
7. There are significant limitations and complications of oral anticoagulant therapy making **LAA** closure an attractive option.
8. In the Prevail trial, the overall efficacy non inferiority was **not** achieved, however non inferiority seven days after the procedure was achieved (18 months follow up).
9. The watchman device has been studied most extensively.
10. The watchman device is indicated as an alternative to warfarin therapy in patient with non-valvular **AF**.
11. Acute procedural related complications are rare. (4%)

12. The four years data from the Protect **AF** trial showed that the watchman device has met the criteria of non inferiority and superiority compared to warfarin for the prevention of stroke, systemic embolisation and cardiovascular death.

Indications for LAAO/ SURGICAL excision:

1. **Surgical** exclusion of **LAA** at the time of mitral valve surgery is a standard practice in many centers.
2. **LAAO** is indicated in (**ESC** 2012 guidelines IIb B):
   a) Patient's refusal of oral anticoagulation.
   b) Relative or absolute contraindication to oral anticoagulation.
   c) Patients with increased risk of bleeding:
      - HAS-BLED score ≥ 3
      - Need for triple anticoagulation therapy. (recent coronary stents, for example)
      - Severe renal failure as a contraindication for **NOACS**.

Complications of LAAO (7%-10%)

1. Cardiac perforation with tamponade. (5%)
2. Air embolism.
3. Development of thrombus on the device. (4%)
4. Stroke. (2%)
5. Device embolisation. (1.5%)
6. Incomplete occlusion of **LAA** with small jet residual flow (14%) which might lead to thrombus formation.

References:

1. Sievert H. et al. Percutaneous Left Atrial Appendage Transcatheter Occlusion to Prevent Stroke. Circulation 2002; 105:1887-9
2. Healey J.S. et al; The LAAOS Pilot Study for Left Atrial Appendage Occlusion during CABG. Am. Heart J. 2005; 150:288-93
3. Holmes D.R. et al. PROTECT AF Trial. Lancet. 2009; 374:534-42
4. Dawson et al, Should Patients with AF Have LAA Exclusion During Cardiac Surgery?. Interact cardiovasc thorac surg. 2010; 10:306-11
5. Park J.W. et al; LAA Closure With AMPLATZER® Cardiac Plug. Catheter Cardiovasc Interv. 2011; 77:700-6
6. 2012 Focused Update of the ESC Guidelines for the Management of Atrial Fibrillation. Europace (2012) 14, 1385-1413
7. Holmes D. et al. The (PREVAIL) Trial. JACC. 2014; 64(1) 1-12
8. Meier B. et al; EHRA/EAPCI Expert Consensus Statement on Catheter- based Left Atrial Appendage Occlusion. Europace 2014; 16; 1397
9. Chugh A etal. ACC, HRS, SCAI Statement on LAA occlusion device. JACC June 29, 2015.

Coarctation of Aorta (CoA)

Key points to remember:

1. **CoA** is considered as part of generalised arteriopathy, and is often associated with diffuse hypoplasia of the aortic arch and isthmus.

2. **Surgical** repair is standard treatment in infants and young children and in patients with suboptimal anatomy with tortuosity and arch hypoplasia.

3. While percutaneous intervention (Stenting) is the standard treatment for adolescents and adults.

4. Intervention (whether surgical or stenting) is indicated in:
    a) Coarctation gradient of more than 20 mmHg. (Class IC)
    b) Coarctation gradient of less than 20 mmHg with hypertension or the presence of significant collaterals. (Class IIa C)
    c) Failure of balloon angioplasty procedure due to aortic recoil.

5. Persistent or recurring hypertension after successful treatment is common and represents a major long-term problem. (30% remain hypertensive).

6. Pregnancy increases the risks of aneurysm formation, dissection, intracerebral haemorrhage and preeclampsia. Therefore, **intervention** may be necessary if blood pressure is poorly controlled.

7. Immediate effect of stenting on blood pressure lowering is excellent.

8. However, there is a lack of evidence regarding late effectiveness concerning the durability of blood pressure lowering.

9. It is uncertain what can be expected in the longer term regarding blood pressure and the occurrence of late complications especially aneurysm formation.

Types of intervention (stenting or surgery)

1. **Stenting** is the first choice in adults with native **CoA**.
2. For recoarctation or residual **CoA**, balloon **angioplasty** with or without stenting, is the treatment of choice.
3. For infants and young children, and patients with sub- optimal anatomy with tortuosity and hypoplasia of aortic arch, **surgical** repair is the treatment of choice.
4. The development of aneurysms as a complication of balloon angioplasty or surgical repair is generally treated with **surgery**. (however, stent **graft** might have a role in the future).

Contraindications of stenting:

1. **Infants** and young children, as there is no suitable size stent which can be dilated in future to an adult- size aorta.
2. **Complex** anatomy and hypoplasia of aortic arch.
3. **Aberrant** origin of head and neck vessels from the aortic arch.

Complications of stenting

Acute complications: (15%)

1. Dissection, rupture. (4%)
2. Stent migration. (5%)
3. Stroke. (<1%)

Late complications:

1. Aortic dissection.
2. Aneurysm formation. (5-8%)
3. Recoarctation. (7%)
4. Stent fracture. (uncommon)
5. Systemic hypertension.

References:

1. Lababidi Z., Neonatal Transluminal Balloon Coarctation Angioplasty. Am. Heat J. 1983; 106; 106:752-3
2. Redington A. et al; Transcatheter Stent Implantation to Treat Aortic Coarctation in Infancy. Br. Heart J. 1993; 69:80-2
3. Cowley C.G. et al; Long- term Randomised Comparison of Balloon Angioplasty and Surgery for Native Coarctation of the Aorta in Childhood. Circulation. 2005; 111:3453
4. Eicken A. et al. The Fate of Systemic Blood Pressure in Patients after Effectively stented coarctation. Eur. Heart J. 2006; 27:1100-5
5. Forbes T.J. Et al; (CCISC) Study. Catheter cardiovasc. interv. 2007; 70:276-85

6. Egan M. et al; Comparing Balloon Angioplasty, Stenting and Surgery in the Treatment of Aortic Coarctation. Cardiovasc ther. 2009; 7:1401-12

7. ESC 2010, Guidelines for the Management of Grown- up Congenital Heart Disease. Baumgartner H. et al; European Heart Journal (2010) 31, 2915-2957

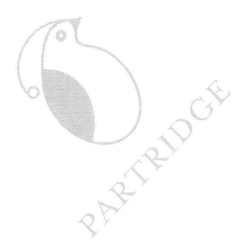

Carotid Artery Stenting (CAS)

Key points to remember:

1. The results of **CAS** are usually influenced by the anatomy of the aortic arch and supra-aortic vessels. While the results of **carotid endarterectomy (CEA)** are influenced by the patient's comorbidities.

2. Conditions leading to increased procedural risks of CAS are:
    a) Age above 70 years.
    b) Severely diseased aortic arch.
    c) Tortuous **CCA** or **ICA**.

3. The stroke risk of intervention in **asymptomatic** patients should not exceed the risk of natural course with medical treatment of carotid stenosis. (1%-3% per year)

4. For **CAS**, the experience of the hospital and operators correlate with the outcomes – the stroke or death rate should not be above **6%** for symptomatic patients, and not above **3%** for asymptomatic ones. Otherwise, revascularisation may have no advantages over medical treatment.

5. The overall result of the CREST trial in symptomatic and asymptomatic patients - showed the primary endpoint of a composite of any stroke, MI or death was similar in **CAS** and **CEA**.

6. However, in the **subgroup** of **symptomatic** patients and patients above the age of **70**, it showed the **superiority** of **CEA** over **CAS**, and also CREST trial has found that stroke has a significant effect on **quality** of life compared to myocardial infarction.

7. The benefit of revascularisation by **CAS** or **CEA** versus modern aggressive medical therapy (antiplatelets, statins, and antihypertensive) has **not** been established for patients with asymptomatic carotid stenosis.

8. In symptomatic patients above the age of 70, the risk of stroke or death is **twofold** higher with **CAS** compared to **CEA**.

   So, **CEA** is **Prefered** in:
   a) Surgically accessible lesions.
   b) Absence of clinically significant cardiac, pulmonary or other diseases increasing the risk of surgery.
   c) No prior ipsilateral endarterectomy.

9. **CAS** is **Prefered** in:
   a) If a carotid lesion is not accessible for surgery. b) In radiation-induced carotid stenosis.
   b) In patients with significant cardiac, pulmonary or other diseases which increase the **risk** of anesthesia and surgery.

10. **CEA** is **not** beneficial for patients with near-occlusion of the carotid artery.

11. Patients with stroke who have persistent disabling neurologic deficits are **unlikely** to benefit from any revascularization (CEA or CAS).

ASA/ACCF/AHA/SCAI) 2011 Guidelines for the Management of Patients with Carotid Disease:

1. **CAS is reasonable over CEA for patients who have**:
   a) Anatomic or medical conditions that increase the risk of surgery.
   b) Radiation-induced restenosis. c) Restenosis after surgery.
   c) Unfavorable neck anatomy.

2. For **asymptomatic** patients with severe non-invasive (70-99%) stenosis, **CEA** should be considered (IIa A) as long as the expected stroke and death rate is less than 3%.

3. Carotid revascularization is **not** recommended for chronic total occlusion, and medical treatment is the **only** practical option.

Summary of the Recommendations for Selecting CEA or CAS: (AHA/ASA) 2014 Guidelines for Stroke Prevention

1. For **symptomatic** patients with severe non-invasive (70-90%) stenosis, **CEA** is recommended.

2. For **symptomatic** patients with moderate (50-69%) stenosis, **CEA** is recommended depending on patient specific factors. (age, sex and comorbidities)

3. **CAS** can be an **alternative** to **CEA** for **symptomatic** patients at an average or low risk of complications associated with stenting if the stenosis is above 70% by non-invasive or 50% by angiography.

Complications of CAS:

1. Carotid sinus reaction: (rare) transient bradycardia, hypotension, asystole, due to stimulation of the carotid baroreceptors.
2. Acute vessel occlusion, due either to severe spasm, dissection, or thrombus formation.
3. Distal embolisation. (0.5-1.5%)
4. Intracranial haemorrhage. (rare)
5. Hyperperfusion syndrome (< 1%), which presents with headache, vomiting, confusion, agitation, seizure and is due to increased perfusion pressure following revascularisation.
6. Contrast induced encephalopathy, which is a transient neurological syndrome which resolves completely in 24 hours.
7. Carotid artery perforation. (0.3%)
8. In-stent restenosis. (< 5%)
9. Stroke. (1.5-5%)

Complications of CEA:

1. Myocardial infarction. (< 2%)
2. Stroke. (0.5-3%)
3. Cerebral hyperperfusion syndrome. (rare)
4. Cervical haematoma.
5. Cranial nerve injury (5%), including hypoglossal, facial and recurrent laryngeal nerves.
6. Wound infections.
7. Carotid restenosis. (2-10%)

CEA compared to CAS has:

1. Superior results in symptomatic patients.
2. Superior results in patients above the age of 70 years.
3. Superior results in asymptomatic patients.
4. Lower incidence of stroke.
5. Lower incidence of distal embolisation
6. Higher incidence of MI.
7. Higher incidence of restenosis

References:

1. Kastrup. et al; Early Outcome of Carotid Angioplasty and Stenting With and Without Cerebral Protection Devices. Stroke. 2003; 34:813-9
2. Yadav J.S. et al; Protected Carotid artery Stenting Versus Endarterectomy in High-risk Patients. N. Eng. J. Med. 2004; 351:1493-501
3. Macdonald S. et al; The evidence of cerebral protection. Analysis and summary of the literature. Eur. J. Radio. 2006; 60:20
4. Mas J.L. (EVA-3S) trial. Lancet Neurol. 2008; 7:885-92
5. Nedeltchev K. et al; Standardised Definitions and Clinical End Points in Carotid Artery and Supra-aortic trunk Revascularisation Trials. Catheter cardiovasc. interv. 2010; 76:333-44
6. Silver F.L. (CREST) trial. Stroke 2011; 42:675
7. Brott T.G. et al., ASA/ACCF/AHA/SCAI guidelines on the management of patients with extracranial carotid and vertebral arteries. J.A.C.C., 57, issue 8, Febr. 2011, e16-e94.
8. Michael Tendera et al; ESC guidelines 2011, on the diagnosis and treatment of peripheral artery disease. Europen H. J. (2011) 32, 2851-2906

9. Van Der Heyden J. et al; High Versus Standard Clopidogrel Dose in Patients Undergoing Carotid Stenting. (IMPACT) trial. J. cardiovasc surg. (Torino) 2013; 54:337

10. Tandros R.O. et al; The effect of statin use on embolic potential during carotid angioplasty and stenting. Ann. Vasc. Surg.2013; 27:96

11. Kernan W.N. et al; AHA/ASA guidelines for the prevention of stroke and TIA. Stroke 2014; 45:2160

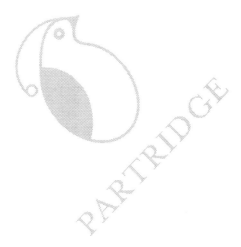

Renal Artery Stenting (RAS)

Causes of Renal Artery Stenosis:

1. Atherosclerosis
2. Fibromuscular dysplasia.
3. Nephroangiosclerosis.(hypertensive injury)
4. Aortorenal dissection.
5. Renal artery vasculitis.
6. Thromboangiitis obliterans.
7. Scleroderma.
8. Trauma.

Key points to remember in patients with renal artery stenosis:

1. Renovascular disease is suspected if there are clinical clues:
   a) Acute elevation of serum creatinine.
   b) Severe hypertension in patients with diffuse systemic atherosclerosis.
   c) Moderate- severe hypertension in patients with recurrent flash pulmonary edema.
   d) Onset of hypertension before the age of 30 and after the age of 55.
   e) Systolic or diastolic abdominal bruit.
   f) Worsening of renal function after administration of **ACI** or **ARB** agent.
   g) Unexplained atrophic kidney.

h) Multivessel coronary artery disease or peripheral artery disease.

2. Revascularisation (stenting or surgery) is reasonable only for patients who have a high likelihood of benefitting from intervention. These conditions (appropriate care criteria for revascularisation) are:

a) **Short** duration of hypertension prior to the diagnosis of renal artery stenosis.

b) **Failure** of optimal medical therapy. c) **Intolerance** to medical therapy.

c) **Deterioration** of renal function.

d) Recurrent **flash** pulmonary edema in patients with normal left ventricle systolic function.

Patients who do not meet any **one** of the above criteria should be treated with **medical therapy** alone.

3. **Not** appropriate care of revascularization:

a) Unilateral, bilateral or solitary kidney with **RAS** and controlled blood pressure and normal renal function.

b) Unilateral, bilateral or solitary kidney with **RAS** and kidney size is < 7 cm.

c) Unilateral, bilateral or solitary kidney with **RAS** and chronic end-stage renal disease.

d) Chronic total occlusion of renal artery.

4. Meta-analysis of the seven **randomised** trials (including STAR, ASTRAL and CORAL) did **not** demonstrate important clinical benefit of stenting over medical treatment, however the CORAL trial did not evaluate those patients who failed optimal medical

therapy, and many patients were **not** eligible for inclusion in the trial, so it did **not** represent **real world** patients.

5. However, the results of stenting from **observational** studies in patients with high-risk subsets showed greater benefit from stenting compared to those patients enrolled in randomised trials.

6. These benefits of stenting are:
    a) Lower mortality.
    b) Lower risk of cardiovascular events.
    c) Lower rate of renal disease progression. d) Decrease in serum creatinine.
    d) Lower incidence of hospitalisation from heart failure.

7. The high-risk subsets of patients are:
    a) Patients with flash pulmonary edema.
    b) Resistant hypertension. (requiring 3 or more drugs)
    c) Chronic renal insufficiency, with creatinine < 3 mg/dl.
    d) d) Acute renal failure.

8. Potential **concerns** of medical treatment alone:
    a) Progression of the stenosis.
    b) Ischemic damage of the affected kidney in the long term.
    c) Impairment of kidney function by inhibiting the protective effect of angiotensin.

9. Revascularisation by **surgery** is indicated only for patients with complex anatomical lesions of the renal artery, not amenable to stenting.

10. The treatment of choice for **fibromuscular** dysplasia is   plain balloon angioplasty and possibly cutting balloon angioplasty with a high possibility of curing the hypertension.

11. The ESC 2011 guidelines consider renal stenting a (Class IIb A) indication.

12. Revascularisation **rarely** cures the hypertension but it might improve the control of blood pressure.

13. Angiographic stenosis of >70% indicates severe stenosis and is hemodynamically significant.

Complications of stenting:

1. Renal artery dissection.
2. Renal artery thrombosis.
3. Renal artery perforation, often needing surgical treatment.
4. Acute kidney injury due either to atheromatous emboli or to contrast agent.
5. Restenosis. (11-17%)

Contraindications to renal stenting:

1. Limited life expectancy.
2. Advanced kidney disease. (creatinine > 3-4 mg/dl)
3. Patients with bleeding diathesis
4. Recent myocardial infarction.
5. Pregnancy.

References:

1. Plouin P.F. et al; Blood Pressure Outcome of Angioplasty in Atherosclerotic Renal Artery Stenosis. The EMMA Study Group. Hypertension. 1998; 31:823-9

2. Van de ven P.J.et al; Arterial Stenting and Balloon Angioplasty in Ostial Atherosclerotic Renovascular Disease. Lancet. 1999; 353:282-6

3. Van Jaarsveld BC et al; The Effect of Balloon Angioplasty on Hypertension in Atherosclerotic Renal Artery Stenosis. N. Eng. J. Med. 2000; 342: 1007-14

4. Sapoval M. et al; GREAT Trial. J. Vasc. Intervene. Rradiool. 2005; 16:1195-202

5. Hirsch A.T. et al; ACC/AHA Guidelines for the Management of Patients with Peripheral Arterial Disease. Circulation. 2006; 113:e463

6. Astral Trial. N. Eng. J. Med. 2009; 361:1953-62

7. Michael Tendera et al; ESC guidelines 2011, on the diagnosis and treatment of peripheral artery disease. Europen H. J. (2011) 32, 2851-2906

8. Cooper C.J. et al. CORAL Trial. N. Eng. J. Med. 2014; 370:13

9. Riaz I.B. et al. Meta- analysis of Revascularisation Versus Medical Therapy for Atherosclerotic Renal Artery Stenosis. Am. J. Cardiol. 2014; 114:116

10. Ritchie J. et al. High-risk Clinical Presentations in Atherosclerotic Renovascular Disease: Prognosis and Response to Renal Artery Revascularisation. Am. J. Kidney. Dis. 2014; 63:186

11. Park S etal. SCAI Expert Consunsus Statement for Renal Artery Stenting Appropriate Use. Catheterisation and Cardiovascular Interventions 84;1163-1171(2014)

Renal Artery Sympathetic Denervation (RSD)

Key points to remember:

1. Resistant hypertension is defined as a blood pressure above 140/90 mmHg despite the use of 3 or 4 anti- hypertensives including diuretics.
2. Several non-blind studies have shown that renal denervation significantly reduces blood pressure in patients with resistant hypertension.
3. The simplicity-HTN 3 trial (blind randomised) failed to demonstrate any benefit after six months.
4. Currently, some centers are performing renal denervation on patients with resistant hypertension with suitable renal artery anatomy. (Renal artery diameter of more than 4 mm with only one artery supplying each kidney).
5. The old concept was RSD is a simple procedure that could be performed with little training by any interventionist, however the new concept that it is recognized as a complex specialized therapy whose success depend on a large number of influencing factors and uncertainties that may not be filled by our current knowledge.
6. It is difficult to standardize treatment recommendations due to different systems and strategies available.
7. Asymmetric and most probably distal renal artery targeting is required to achieve effective ablation.

8. Maximum procedural efficacy would mean the achievement of ablation in all four quadrants and the whole circumference of both renal arteries.
9. There appear to be a dose response dependency between the number of ablations and the efficacy of ablation
10. The feasibility, the need, and the consequences of treating small renal arteries < 4mm remained to be clarified.
11. The lack of procedural markers of immediate success remains the major unmet need.
12. **RSD** did not show untoward effect on renal functions and no orthostatic hypotension.
13. Better results are obtained with deeper and circumferential ablation, and distal ablation in the renal artery branches.
14. Avoid ostial ablation as it may lead to aortic dissection.
15. Avoid areas of atheroma and stenosis.
16. **RSD** is currently a Class II b indication.

Complications

1. Renal artery spasm.
2. Renal artery dissection.
3. Renal artery stenosis.
4. Aortic dissection.

Possible future applications

Patients with increased sympathetic activations:

1. Obstructive sleep apnoea.
2. Polycystic ovary syndrome,

3. Chronic heart failure.
4. Metabolic syndrome.

References:

1. Krum H. et al; Catheter- based Renal Sympathetic Denervation for Resistant Hypertension. Lancet. 2009; 373:1275-81
2. Esler M.D. et al; (the simplicity HTN2 trial) Lancet.2010: 376:1903-9
3. Krum H. et al; Catheter- based Renal Sympathetic Denervation for Resistant Hypertension: Durability of Blood pressure Reduction out to 24 Months. Hypertension. 2011; 57:911-7
4. Witkowski A. et al; Effects of Renal Sympathetic Denervation on Blood Pressure, Sleep Apnea Course and Glycemic Control in Patients With Resistant Hypertension and Sleep Apnea. Hypertension. 2011; 58:559-65
5. Bhatt D.L et al; (Simplicity HTN-3 trial): A Controlled Trial of Renal Denervation for Resistant Hypertension. N. Eng. J. Med. 2014; 370:1393
6. Euro PCR, Paris, may 2015.